HYDRATE RIGHT!

The Effective Way To Drink Water

By

Dr. Lesley Ike

This book is dedicated to: Clara and Mari-Joyce Dansby, my rocks that I silently watch and learn from since we met. Thank you for paving the pathway with love yet teaching strength. To Rod, Reggie, Sean, Tony, Chris and Timmy, the men I love more than life itself and without whom I could not be the princess. To my dad who transitioned way too soon, but his wisdom and words still flow to me. To my grandparents whom I was able to spend my summers with and gain so much wisdom and love from. To Leola Ransfer whom I never had the honor to meet, but could have, had she had this knowledge. The numerous patients who have changed their lives just by properly hydrating. My family who will always be a part of every journey in which I embark.

Table of Contents

Introduction

DRINK YOUR WATER!!!

So many people seem to keep reiterating to us that we need to drink our water. We have all heard this from our doctors, our nutritionist, our coaches, at the gym and all our lives from our parents and older family members.

BUT

Why is it that no one has ever taught us how to drink our water? How is this the most abundant resource and the consistency of our body make up are water, yet we are hardly ever told how to drink water properly. We are just told to drink it. We are even told the amount we should drink a day, but we are rarely, if at all told how to properly drink water.

This book will show you the simple, common-sense way to drink water which will keep you hydrated the entire day.

This is a simple and easy book to carry around and pass out to friends and family members to keep them on the proper hydration path, because our lives depend on it. This is the one activity we need to do every day of our lives for the rest of our lives, so take a few minutes, read this book, and bring your body back to its proper hydration state. Your body will thank you later.

It should also be noted that this booklet is not written to highlight my intelligence, but just the opposite. This book was written so a ten-year-old can translate it into their native tongue to share with their parents or grandparents who do not speak the English language. This is also written for the school children who are starting out on their quest for good health and will not have to translate medical terms, but just learn how to properly hydrate from a firm foundation.

PART I: Changing Old Habits And Traditions

I have noticed that people daily do not drink enough water if any at all. I see constantly, people carry water around in their refillable containers or plastic bottle and still do not drink enough water throughout the day for their body to properly function. People whom I have spoken with have been told to drink about two liters per day, yet with drinking this amount of water, so many people still are severely dehydrated. A good amount of my patients has shared with me that they drink a gallon of water a day, I say to them, "No you do not, because if you did, you would not be so dry. The people just laugh at me, in laughing at themselves, but say, "No, I really do drink that much water in a day." I then say to them, "If you are drinking that much water in a day and you are still dehydrated, then you are drinking water wrong, and you are probably urinating all day long as well." They usually laugh and admit that they in fact do spend too much time in the bathroom urinating

Sadly, with my patients, the excessive urinating moves them to stop drinking water all together, because they do not want to spend time in the bathroom, and it interrupts their day. This is a big issue I explain to them, because if their body is seventy to seventy five percent water and no water is going into their system, where will the water you need to survive come from? The answers I get are, from their coffee or tea they drink every morning, from the foods they eat, from their pops/sodas, or from the juices they drink throughout the day. Well, even with all of those, that still is not enough water to keep your muscles, bones, sinews, eyes, hair, skin, nails, bowels…moist. I ask again, where is your body getting the necessary water from to remain properly hydrated? My patients, when asked this question look at me as if I have three heads or am asking them a trick question. So, we are going to take a journey into proper hydration, and the proper way to drink water.

Chapter One: Water And Body Basics

My patients are told that their body consists of seventy-to-seventy five percent of water. Though with this knowledge, they still do not give their bodies the proper amount of water daily. They have even been told to drink a percentage of their body weight in water, patients are even told to drink two to three liters per day. These may be all good, but people still have the problem of the need to constantly use the bathroom. Everyone knows they need water to survive, but no one takes this life necessity serious enough. Let us investigate the different body parts to determine just how important water really is.

The human brain is 80-85% water

Kidneys are 80-85% water

The human heart is 75-80% water

Lungs are 75-80% water

Muscles contain 70-75% water

The human liver is 80-85% water

Skin which is the largest human organ is 70-75% water

Blood consists of 83-85% water

Bones are 20-25% water

Teeth are 8-10% water

When I was in school learning about the human body, though we were given these figures to learn and know, it never really dawned on me how important water really is to the body. Now that I have treated so many patients that are severely dehydrated, I recall the classes I have had in the past to try to help them. I also share with my patients that water is necessary to produce saliva to get the digestive process activated. Water is vital for the brain for hormones and neurotransmitter's proper function and production. Water regulates body temperatures as antifreeze does for one's car. Water flushes out bodily wastes and as we get older, we find out that water lubricates our joints.

The human body is a highly intelligent computer/machine, when it is properly lubricated, like a well-oiled car, it will function smoothly and will function for the long haul. What is interesting is that the human body has a mechanism that will signal your brain when it needs water. When we are thirsty, this mechanism is letting us know that our bodies need water. If we answer the signal to drink water, our bodies can function properly as they were designed to do. When we ignore this signal, our bodies will naturally stop sending the signal due to lack of response and then the body will go into survival mode, because the only thing the human body knows how to do is to keep us alive. If we do not help it out, it will do all it can to keep our blood flowing, to keep our lungs, heart, brain, and all organs properly functioning, because this is all it knows. Therefore, it is so important to listen to our bodies. When we wait until we are thirsty, we are already dehydrated. I remember growing up, a mother figure to me would always say," You need to eat something." I would respond, "I am not hungry." She would say, "You do not eat because you are hungry, you eat so you don't get hungry." The same holds true with drinking water. You drink water, so you do not become thirsty. My greatest advice would be to listen to your body and take the necessary actions to answer every time it feels, senses, or is moved to do something. It is always right. Listen to your body now because the body always wins.

Also, I would add, when the weather changes like it does in south Florida for our "two weeks" of winter. When your body is accustomed to one hundred percent of humidity, as soon as the air cools and dries out, just know that you will need to intake more water to compensate for the lack of humidity your body is used to the other remaining weeks of the year. When it is cold and dry, please drink more water, because your body is adjusting to the change, but we are not keeping up with the change our bodies are going through. During our "winters" in south Florida, I notice an increase in back pains, neck pains, joint pains, dry eyes and more, only because our bodies are trying to stay alive and we just want to go on with our daily routine, and what patients will state during these times, is how thirsty they have been lately. I once again give my hydration lecture to them and tell them to listen, to slow down and listen to their bodies.

From my years of practice, I notice the similarities throughout the spectrum of patients. All in which had the common denominator of dehydration. The main one is lower back pain from people who have never had a fall nor were in an accident or any other back injury. It is also noted that the back pain comes and goes, how their back hurts when they roll out of the bed, how as they start moving the back pain goes away or is diminished, and how this happens in every age group, not just in the elderly. I started watching the different signs and symptoms of my patients and noticed that knee pain, shoulder pain, neck pain, joint pain, dry eyes, dizziness, some cases of tinnitus and swellings of the body were rooted in dehydration. All these individuals were looking to get rid of the symptoms, but no one was addressing the root of their problems. I would be told by my patients that they tried everything, but nothing is working. When they returned for the same treatment, I sought out and prayed for an answer to give my patients hope and relief for their ailments. So, through prayer and different personal tests and trials, I produced my hydration protocol. This is the protocol I share with all my patients and anyone I see with the conditions or symptoms in which I have been able to study. A great teacher for me was watching my pets and their water drinking habits. I noticed that they were frequently at their water bowl taking a couple of sips, so to say, of water. I would think, this is their instinct, why am I not doing the same and I need water just as much as they do. I then began to listen to my body instead of just busying myself to avoid drinking water and just started drinking water.

Chapter Two: How Do I Effectively And Properly Hydrate?

This is the million-dollar, life changing question.

To date, I have had four patients who were scheduled to have lower back surgery performed. I asked them to give me three weeks to properly hydrate them and see if a surgery is needed. These four brave souls trusted me enough to see if I was telling the truth about hydration or not and are still to this day happy they listened, because all four of them remain surgery free and are still thriving in their health.

To begin with I teach them about how the human body processes water and how they are drinking water wrong to begin with, are not drinking enough water, and have not been drinking water properly for years. This is what I share with all my patients now because the minor aches and pains felt in their bodies, can be alleviated if only they were properly hydrated.

I ask my patients to make a fist, they all make a fist, and I ask them to look at their fist, in reply, they all look at their fist. I go on to explain to them that their fist is about the size of their kidney and is about four to five ounces, depending on how big or small the individual is. I must give them a visual so they can grasp the amount of water to properly drink. I go on to tell them that their kidney can only hold about four to five ounces at a time to filter through our system. I say to them, you cannot put a twelve-ounce bottle of water in a four-ounce kidney and expect it to function properly. If one wishes to have their kidney function properly, I suggest drinking four ounces of water every thirty minutes, which is about four to five swallows of water. I ask my patients to measure out four or five ounces and count how many swallows it is for them and use that as your benchmark. This way the kidney can properly filter the water as it was designed to do and the water will reach the necessary organs, vessels, sinews, joints, bones, etcetera. I let them know that anything over four or five ounces, your body will think of it as excess and waste and spit it out as waste and therefore most people spend so much time in the bathroom urinating throughout the day.

If the intake of water is four to five ounces every thirty minutes, it will properly hydrate the body and the need to use the bathroom is diminished because the water is being effectively used in the body. The color of urine of a properly hydrated person should be a lite straw color. This will indicate that the kidneys are filtering properly. Urine that is too dark, your body is in dire need of water. If it is clear, the kidneys are not filtering, but just pushing the water through.

When I do this hydration protocol, I use the bathroom four times the entire day, and I stay hydrated. Before I started testing this out on myself, I would have to use the bathroom two to three times an hour, I would rush into restaurants, stores, amusement parks, museums and the first thing I would ask was, "Where are the restrooms?" I really did not enjoy going out because of this bathroom issue I was dealing with. I slowed down to analyze all that I have studied, and this is what I produced. Something so simple that has changed my life and the lives of my patients and their families.

Along with the water intake every thirty minutes, I add a little Himalayan pink salt, Kosher salt, or sea salt, lemons, limes or both lemons and limes. This is the fastest and safest sports drink for hydration you can easily make at home without all the sugars that most sports drinks have. Here is a simple drink that will hydrate you and replace electrolytes that are lost in the process of sweating and urinating.

If you feel you are hydrated and get muscle cramps at night, or if you work out, or play in a sport as I do, I continue my water regimen and drink pickle juice. Yes! Pickle juice! Pickle juice,

(Dill Pickles) will super hydrate you as well as take muscle cramps and pains away. People ask me, "Isn't that too much salt?" I say, "When you are working out, what are you losing? Even daily, without working out, what is your body excreting? Urine is a mixture of water, salts and urea, perspiration is salt and water. So, daily if we are not replenishing the salts and water, where are they going to come from?

People ask me, "Will all of that salt and water make my ankles swell?" All my patients that have come in with swollen ankles and feet, have properly hydrated and the swelling went down. The patients I know that have congestive heart failure will have a different water protocol than the norm. After a thorough intake and exam, it is easy to assess who needs what, so please do not self-diagnose yourself.

I have had a patient who had swelling up to their thighs and were placed on water pills. I explained to her that their body is holding onto water, because you are not giving your body enough water to survive, so it went into survival mode and stored the water, like a camel does, to keep it functioning properly. This patient could barely walk when she came into the clinic and during the intake, she admitted that she has not had a drink of water in a long time. I showed her how to drink water and treated her twice a week and in three weeks her legs were her normal size, and she was able to walk again, she was also taken off about three different medications because she no longer needed them. She hated the taste of water and just would not drink it because of the taste. I had her add the pink salt and fruits and vegetables to her water and to eat the foods she put in her water. She put in her favorite fruits and vegetables and is enjoying water for the first time in her life and her health has drastically improved.

I have another patient who had bone pain, joint pain, constant cramping of muscles, and was barely walking when he walked in my office. He had a condition of internal heat and wind, and he too, was on a plethora of medications. He came to the office once a week for six months and with every treatment I would make him a glass of my personal hydration drink to drink. On a couple of occasions, I would make him a gallon to take home to make sure he would drink it. As time went on, his posture straightened up, he no longer complained about aches and pains, his skin cleared up, his wrinkles filled in, his blood pressure regulated and the dietary changes I put him on as well as the hydration protocol, helped him get back on the golf course, and he has never been happier. His wife is even happier because the two of them can do things together again. This patient told me that his primary doctor told him to keep doing what he is doing, because it is working, and he was taken off many of his prescription medications as well.

Another patient wanted to remove the deep line in her glabella area. She started the hydration protocol and with weekly facial acupuncture, the line between her eyes was raised and leveled with the rest of her skin. She stated that her family kept accusing her of getting Botox or fillers in her forehead, but she took the safest route that will last, and new injections would not need to be repeated. She thought she would never get rid on the line in her forehead, now she cannot stop smiling and telling her story of how acupuncture and drinking water ridded her of facial lines.

Along with the hydration protocol, I would recommend starting a routine of daily and nightly facial moisturizing. Keep your skin that is exposed to the elements protected with a moisturizer to protect your skin as well as keeping your cells hydrated. I use natural oils produced from the earth on my own skin, because the ingredients are minimal. Whichever moisturizer you choose, please read the ingredients on the jar or bottle, because some of the ingredients may be harmful to your skin, or your health.

These are just examples of how hydration can change lives. I think I could author a book on the different testimonies from patients on how a steady, constant, intake of water has changed their lives. Please keep in mind that these are results based on my patients, their intake, and our conversation. It is always wise to consult your physician before making health changes with which you are not familiar. Also, use your common sense and listen to your body. You know you better than any doctor, so listen to your body as only you can do.

Chapter Three: Hydrating Foods

Food is medicine!

I should say, real foods are medicine. In a handful of countries, the people are eating genetically modified foods, foods with chemicals or hormones in them, and foods with additives and preservatives added to them. We are not speaking of these foods. Real food which are not altered by humans have been serving as medicine since the beginning of time. Chinese medicine, which I have studied, the herbs and herbal formulas are all based on nature, and other cultures which use nature as medicine have been doing such for thousands of years with tremendous results. I say all of this to share with you the foods that are excellent for hydration, in their purest forms are medicine as well. There are foods that can be added to this list, but these are prominent in the area in which I currently live and are in abundance in the grocery stores.

Strawberries consist of about 91% water

Watermelon consists of about 92%water

Cantaloupe consists of about 90% water

Peaches consists of about 89% water

Oranges consists of about 88% water

Cucumbers consists of about 95% water

Lettuce consists of about 96% water

Zucchini consists of about 94% water

Celery consists of about 95% water

Tomatoes consists of about 94% water

Bell Peppers consist of about 92% water

Cauliflower consists of about 92% water

Cabbage consists of about 92% water

Grapefruit consists of about 88% water

Coconut water consists of about 95% water

Again, there are more foods that consist of a high percentage of water, these are just the ones that I picked out. Even with all of these and more water filled foods, it is still necessary to take a steady constant intake of water itself throughout the day.

Chapter Four: Conversations With The Water Doc

I am going to share conversations that I deal with every day from different patients. My patients end up laughing at me and the conversations but go home and try the water protocol, all to come back to tell me of their positive changes their bodies have gone through. I hope you get as much of a laugh out of these as I give my patients and myself.

After teaching my patients how to properly drink water…

Patient: I hate water, I just cannot see myself drinking that all day long.

Me: You really do not hate water, because your entire body is comprised of water. You just hate that it is not sweet and has no flavor.

So, I suggest that you put fruit and cucumbers in the water with a pinch of pink salt, this way you will properly hydrate as well as get the phytochemicals from the fruits and vegetables used in your water mixture.

Patient: If I drink like that all day, I will pee all day long, I am not going to do that, because I do not have time to be in the bathroom all day long.

Me: No, in fact, if you drink four ounces every thirty minutes, you will urinate fewer times throughout the day because the water is finally reaching your skin, muscles, tendons, ligaments, brain, hair, nails… and you will be properly hydrated, not to mention your wrinkles will start to fill in as well.

Do not tell me you cannot do this because if you were at a party, you could down two bottles of wine or six beers in two hours, or less without any problems and these will dehydrate you faster than anything, but you cannot drink a little water every thirty minutes?

Patient: Cannot stop laughing

Patient: Well, I do not drink alcohol!

Me: Well, the same with coffee and pops/sodas! You have no problem downing twenty ounces of coffee or soda in thirty minutes or less and you don't even bat an eye, so you tell me you cannot drink four ounces of water?

Patient: Even more laughter

Patient: You are right doc when you put it that way, I know I can do better with my water intake.

Me: I know you can, just try it for three weeks and let me know how your body transforms and let me know about the people who ask you what you are doing because you look so great. Then when you get all these compliments coming your way, you will smile inside and say, "Thanks Doc!" Then I want you to come back and tell me all the stories.

Patient: Doc you tell me all these things about water, but how is water going to help me with all the pain I have? It cannot be that easy.

Me: It really is that easy, we just complicate everything. If you think about your joints, there is cartilage between your bones, right? Well, think about a dry sponge sitting on the edge of your sink, it is shriveled up and hard to move, but once you add water to it, it expands, it is flexible and pliable. The same with your cartilage, it shrinks and shrivels up when not properly hydrated, this brings your bones closer together, pressing the cartilage down and causing pain and inflammation. When properly hydrated, the cartilage expands and cushions the bones and acts as shock absorbers for your bones as cartilage was designed to do, and the pain and inflammation goes away. If you go years without proper hydration, your cartilage will degenerate and your bones touch and when this happens, the only thing left to do is surgery, because the cartilage is completely gone. That is why I push you to hydrate now, because over time, this will be the outcome, because the body always wins. You can neglect it now, but twenty to thirty years from now, you will wish you went the extra mile to do the little menial things.

Patient: Yes, you are right, I never looked at it that way, but now it makes sense. I must do better in drinking my water.

On a much more personal occasion where I saw with my own eyes how proper hydration is vital to so many ailments. After the funeral of my father, a family member had trouble walking and their legs cramped up so severely that they were screaming. I immediately performed acupuncture on this individual and had my brother rush to get pickle juice and a hydration drink. We had her drink this for the next 45 minutes then started giving her water every 30 minutes and the pain went away, cramping went away, and she was feeling like herself once again.

With another family member, she kept having dizzy spells and kept passing out and the doctors could not find any reason as to why this was happening. I kept telling her to hydrate, this is all you need, and the dizziness will go away. Well, as you suspected, she did not listen and fell where she was getting physical therapy. She was administered two IV's and has not had a dizzy, or fainting spell since, because she started hydrating.

Conclusion

I am often asked, "Doc, is it really that simple? I reply, "Yes, it really **IS** that simple!"

God made hydrating so simple, but our fast-paced life has complicated it. We sometimes feel like drinking water throughout the day is a burden because we must stop what we are doing just to take in a little water. I would suggest going back to basics because the body always wins. You can either hydrate now or deal with the aches, pains, and degenerations that your body will go through as you age if you do not hydrate. Just try this protocol for 6 weeks, do not cheat, because you will be only cheating yourself, but try it and let me know how this hydration protocol has changed your life. It has for sure changed mine and my patients who continue to do it. Make it a lifestyle change and watch how your life changes for the better.

Sadly, the days and times we live in today, we are not trained to do the proper things for our health. We quickly run to the doctor to get a pain pill, injection, or as drastic as a surgery instead of doing the simple things as drinking a constant intake of water daily to remain hydrated. We look for the quick and easy fix instead of what our bodies really need. I am glad that I am experiencing patients that are looking for solutions outside of pills and surgery, this happens to be one of the easiest life changes that can answer a tremendous amount of ailments, if properly administered.

Please just remember a steady intake of water is what your body needs. Do not chug the entire glass of water, or bottle of water to check that activity off because your doctor suggested you drink more water. Hydration is not an activity you check off daily to say you did it, hydration is a necessity for life, for the rest of your life.

"When the solutions are simple, God is answering."

…Albert Einstein

Acknowledgments

There are so many people I would like to thank for encouraging me to put this information in writing, my patients who have tried my hydration protocol and have had such life changing results. My dear friend Jackie De Los Santos who transitioned while I was writing this booklet, but while on this plane, she was my biggest fan and encourager to follow any dream that comes to my heart. To the patients who have taken time to take this advice and change their lives. To my friends who remained even while I was in hermit mode to get this finished before the year ended. To my brothers and sisters in the Lord who have kept me in prayer and continue to keep me in prayer as I traverse through this journey. I have great thanks to my Heavenly Father who has given me this knowledge to teach to my patients and share with the world, who in parts of my life is showing me to go back to basics to find your answers. Big thanks for everyone who takes the time to read this, apply it to their lives and continue in it for the rest of their lives. May you all be blessed in all that you do from this point on.

About the Author

Dr. Lesley Ike

Dr. Lesley was born in England, the only daughter of an Airforce Captain/Dentist, and mother who obtained her master's in music was a renowned teacher; raised Lesley and her three brothers in Ohio, where she was an exceptional athlete in volleyball, basketball, and softball, or any sport that crossed her path. Lesley also played the violin for 10 years, but her love for sports is what moved her in the direction to learn about the human body.

Lesley attended the Cincinnati College of Mortuary Science where she received her bachelor's degree in Mortuary Science and practiced in Cincinnati, Ohio. In this field, Lesley was one of the best embalmers and was known for her facial reconstruction and restorative art in which she performed.

After different career successes, Lesley did not feel fulfilled in her destiny, so Lesley attended the Atlantic Institute of Oriental Medicine in Fort Lauderdale, Florida where she was on the dean's list and received her master's in Acupuncture and Chinese Medicine, as well as obtaining her bachelor's degree in Nutritional science. She then went on to study in Shanghai China at the Shuguang hospital, which is affiliated with Shanghai University and is the medical, educational and research center of TCM (Traditional Chinese Medicine) in Asia. In China she studied with the Masters of TCM and honed in her skills in Gynecology, Gastroenterology, Nephrology, TuiNa, Herbology, Pain Management, Sports Medicine, and other courses in which she excelled in.

She decided to become an acupuncturist because she felt her calling was to the profession. Lesley believes that acupuncture enhances people's lives mentally, physically, emotionally & spiritually. Through the past few years, Lesley has helped over fifty women become pregnant who believed would never have babies. This, she says, makes her profession worth It all. Her intentions were to focus on sports medicine, but life took a turn and directed her into becoming "The Baby Maker" as mothers have called her, and "The Water Doctor."

Most people who have experienced getting treatments by Lesley have said that her treatments go far beyond needles and are life changing, spiritual experiences. This could attribute to Lesley's love for people and her profession. Lesley takes her time to get to know her patients and spends time with them and is always available for all who call upon her. Lesley is known for doing comedy acupuncture, for during a session, her gift of comedy sometimes surfaces and has her patients laughing so much that they do not realize she has finished needling them. Laughter is the best medicine and Lesley knows that having people laugh, she is kickstarting their healing session. With every session, you will feel the love Lesley has for life, people and for her profession. You will also get her hydration lecture and will think of her with every drink of water in which you ingest.